CHAIR YOGA FOR MEN OVER 50

Low Impact Fitness Exercise for seniors to build strength, boost Flexibility, gain balance and achieve weight Loss with less Effort

Clair L. Marshall

TABLE OF CONTENT

INTRODUCTION

Meet Thomas, a guy in his early fifties who is dealing with the unavoidable impacts of aging. The once-bright vitality that distinguished his youth appeared to fade, replaced by recurrent hip pains, a nagging soreness in his back, and a pervasive sensation of overall bodily frailty.

Thomas, like many of his friends, attributed his problems to the normal course of aging and his sedentary lifestyle.

However, everything changed for Thomas when he came upon a book that would serve as his road map to fresh vitality—specifically geared for men over 50.

The book not only cleared up misunderstandings about yoga but also introduced him to the notion of chair yoga, which promised comfort without the intimidation of complicated positions.

As Thomas read through the pages of this transforming book, he discovered a wealth of information about adapting conventional yoga techniques to the confines of a chair.

The book functioned as a complete guidebook, providing explicit instructions on motions and stretches that targeted the specific regions where Thomas felt difficulty.

More than just an exercise routine, chair yoga has evolved into a comprehensive approach to well-being that integrates physical and mental wellbeing.

With fresh motivation, Thomas applied the book's precepts to his daily life. The chair became his haven, where he gradually regained control of his body and relieved the recurring aches that had become unpleasant friends. Thomas found that constant practice not only strengthened his core and improved his flexibility but also increased his overall energy levels.

The narrative of Thomas is one of change and tenacity, demonstrating the transforming impact of chair yoga for men over 50. Today, Thomas not only moves with greater physical ease, but he also greets each day with a renewed feeling of vigor.

His path demonstrates the importance of tailoring health practices to individual circumstances and the significant impact such changes can have on quality of life, particularly for individuals entering their senior years.

Chapter 1: What is Chair Yoga ?

Chair yoga is a moderate type of yoga that involves performing classic yoga postures while seated on a chair or utilizing the chair for support.

This technique is especially good for people with restricted mobility, elders, and those recuperating from ailments.

 The major purpose of chair yoga is to make yoga's advantages more accessible to a wider audience while also fostering physical, mental, and emotional well-being.

Chair yoga aims to improve flexibility, strength, and balance. Participants practice modified versions of traditional yoga positions, including twists, stretches, and gentle twists, while sitting comfortably. The chair functions as a steady support, allowing those with mobility difficulties to engage and gradually gain strength.

Aside from the physical advantages, chair yoga promotes focus and breath awareness. Participants are urged to focus on their breath, which promotes relaxation and reduces tension.

This characteristic of chair yoga makes it ideal for people who suffer from chronic pain, arthritis, or other ailments that make conventional yoga difficult.

Chair yoga classes frequently include meditation and guided relaxation, which promotes inner peace and mental clarity.

Chair yoga's accessibility makes it appropriate for a wide range of locations, including businesses, community centers, and senior living institutions. It is easily adaptable to varied fitness levels and physical talents.

One of the primary benefits of chair yoga is its inclusiveness. It allows people who might otherwise feel excluded from typical yoga courses to reap the overall advantages of the practice.

Furthermore, chair yoga may be easily integrated into everyday routines, providing a handy option for people to improve their general well-being.

Chair yoga is a dynamic and inclusive practice that extends the many advantages of conventional yoga to people who have physical limitations.

Chair yoga, which incorporates conscious movement, breathwork, and relaxation methods, provides a comprehensive approach to increasing physical health, lowering stress, and improving overall quality of life.

Understanding the Benefits of Chair Yoga

Chair yoga is a moderate and accessible kind of yoga that has various advantages, particularly for men over 50.

This practice modifies basic yoga postures to be performed while sitting or supported by a chair, making it an excellent choice for anyone with mobility concerns or those looking for a less demanding type of exercise.

One of the primary benefits of chair yoga is its potential to increase flexibility. As men age, their joints may become less elastic, resulting in stiffness.

Chair yoga uses moderate stretches to target different muscle groups, improving range of motion and flexibility without putting undue pressure on the body.

Beyond flexibility, chair yoga improves strength. Many postures use core muscles, which are essential for stability and balance. Strengthening these muscles can help reduce falls, which are a significant concern among older people.

Furthermore, chair yoga encourages good posture, which helps to relieve back pain and discomfort caused by extended sitting.

Another benefit of chair yoga is improved mental health. The practice focuses on mindfulness and deep breathing, which reduce tension and promote relaxation.

Men over 50 frequently encounter particular pressures, such as retirement or health difficulties, and chair yoga offers a comprehensive strategy for addressing these issues.

Chair yoga has cardiovascular advantages as well. While the exercise is low-impact, the combination of flowing motions and regulated breathing can benefit heart health.

This is especially important for older people trying to maintain or improve their cardiovascular fitness without engaging in strenuous activities.

Furthermore, chair yoga is accessible and adaptive. It covers a wide range of fitness levels and is easily adaptable to individual requirements and talents.

This makes it a good choice for guys over 50 who are coping with specific health issues or recuperating from injuries.

Chair yoga is a diverse and effective exercise for guys over 50. It focuses on physical, mental, and emotional well-being, offering a complete approach to sustaining health and vitality in older life.

Tailoring Yoga Practices for Men Over 50

Yoga is a flexible practice that may be adapted to meet the unique needs of men over 50, boosting physical health, emotional well-being, and flexibility.

As people age, it becomes increasingly important to adapt yoga practices to meet changing bodies and potential health issues.

First, concentrate on easy positions that increase flexibility and joint mobility. Incorporate motions that target stiffness-prone regions, including the spine, hips, and shoulders.

Poses like Cat-Cow, moderate twists, and sitting stretches are ideal for maintaining or improving range of motion.

Standing postures such as the warrior series and tree pose can help you gain strength and balance. These not only increase muscle strength but also improve stability, lowering the chance of falls, a major issue among the elderly.

Props like blocks or a chair can be used to provide additional support while emphasizing appropriate alignment.

Breathing exercises, or pranayama, are vital for general health. Deep belly breathing, alternate nostril breathing, and mindful breath awareness can help reduce tension and promote relaxation. Mind-body connection is essential for mental clarity and emotional resilience.

Because cardiovascular health is critical, consider including dynamic sequences like sun salutations. These sequences not only increase heart rate but also provide full-body exercise, improving cardiovascular fitness and endurance. However, adjust the tempo to accommodate different fitness levels, guaranteeing a safe and fun experience.

When teaching yoga to guys over the age of 50, adaptability is essential. Recognize any pre-existing health concerns or limits, and adjust the poses accordingly. Consultation with a healthcare practitioner is recommended, particularly for people with chronic health problems.

Yoga techniques for men over 50 need a careful combination of flexibility, strength, balance, and awareness. Customizing practices to suit physical changes while prioritizing general health provides a long-term and productive yoga practice.

Chapter 2: The Foundations of Chair Yoga

Chair yoga is an accessible and effective practice, particularly for men over 50 who may have physical restrictions or issues.

The principles of chair yoga are based on modifying conventional yoga poses to be practiced while seated, with a chair providing support and stability.

This adjustment makes yoga more accessible and inclusive for people with mobility challenges, ensuring that everyone can reap the many physical and emotional benefits of this ancient practice.

The fundamental goal of chair yoga is to increase flexibility, strength, and balance without putting undue strain on joints. Gentle stretches, regulated movements, and deep breathing exercises are essential components for improving circulation and general well-being.

Chair yoga's sitting nature removes the need for difficult transitions, making it ideal for anyone with limited mobility or recovering from injuries.

Chair yoga can help men over 50 maintain and improve their physical fitness. It treats typical aging concerns, such as stiffness and limited range of motion, by gently stimulating muscles and increasing joint mobility.
The practice helps to alleviate back discomfort, improve posture, and strengthen core muscles, all of which contribute to a higher quality of life.

Furthermore, chair yoga has advantages beyond the physical realm, providing a space for mental relaxation and stress relief.

Mindful breathing and meditation techniques used in chair yoga sessions assist in relaxing the mind, reducing anxiety, and increasing attention.

As men mature, the value of overall well-being becomes more apparent, making chair yoga an excellent practice for nurturing both body and mind.

Chair yoga is easy to include in a regular practice and doesn't take much time, making it ideal for those with hectic schedules.

Whether at home or in a communal environment, chair yoga's versatility means that anyone may reap its benefits without the need for specific equipment or a large practice area.

Chair yoga for men over 50 is based on adaptation, simplicity, and a comprehensive approach to physical and mental well-being.

Individuals who practice this modified style of yoga can improve their flexibility, strength, and balance while developing a sense of inner serenity and resilience.

Exploring Proper Posture and Alignment

Proper posture and alignment are critical components for sustaining general health and well-being, particularly for people over 50 who practice chair yoga.

Adopting the proper sitting position may have a substantial influence on many aspects of health, from lowering muscular strain to improving pulmonary function.

First and foremost, when doing chair yoga, individuals should keep their spines neutral. Sit with your back straight and shoulders relaxed, supporting the spine's natural curvature.
This not only relieves strain on the lower back but also improves circulation and digestion.

Furthermore, it is critical to maintain proper head and neck alignment. Keep the head aligned with the spine and prevent leaning forward or backward.

This not only minimizes neck strain but also promotes good breathing, resulting in a sensation of tranquility and focus during chair yoga sessions.

Paying attention to joint alignment is especially important for adults over the age of 50. Make sure your hips and knees are at 90-degree angles to provide stability and avoid pain.

Place both feet level on the floor to equally distribute weight and lessen the likelihood of lower back discomfort.

When practicing chair yoga, it is critical to be careful of the shoulders and arms. Relax the shoulders and allow them to naturally descend while keeping the arms close to your body. This reduces upper-body strain while also improving energy flow throughout the exercise.

Using focused breathing methods is another important part of maintaining appropriate posture during chair yoga.

Deep, diaphragmatic breathing will increase lung capacity and oxygenate the body, increasing relaxation and lowering tension.

Exploring appropriate posture and alignment in chair yoga for men over 50 is about more than just physical comfort; it's also about developing a holistic feeling of well-being.

By implementing these concepts throughout your practice, you may benefit from the many advantages of chair yoga while also promoting your general health and longevity.

Breath Awareness Techniques for Relaxation

Breath awareness methods are essential for achieving relaxation, and they are especially effective for males over the age of 50 who do chair yoga.

As people age, pressures mount, affecting their physical and mental health. Incorporating attentive breathing into a chair yoga exercise may greatly improve relaxation and general health.

Begin by settling into a comfortable sitting posture in the chair, maintaining correct spinal alignment.

Close your eyes lightly, focusing on the natural rhythm of your breath. Inhale deeply through your nose, extending your chest and belly, before gently exhaling through pursed lips. Concentrate on the sensation of the breath entering and leaving your body.

Introduce a counting method to help you concentrate and manage your breathing. Inhale for four counts, hold for two, then exhale for six.

This careful and controlled technique helps to coordinate breath and movement, promoting a sensation of serenity.

Explore diaphragmatic breathing, which emphasizes diaphragmatic expansion rather than shallow chest breathing. Place one hand on your chest, the other on your abdomen.

Inhale deeply, feeling your abdomen lift, then exhale completely, experiencing the gradual fall.

This approach improves relaxation by engaging the parasympathetic nervous system.

In addition, practice alternate nostril breathing, also known as Nadi Shodhana. Close your eyes and alternately block one nostril with your thumb and ring finger while inhaling and exhaling through the other.

This practice helps to balance the brain's left and right hemispheres, increasing mental clarity and calmness.

Consistently incorporating these breath awareness methods into chair yoga exercises for men over 50 can help to reduce stress, increase attention, and boost general well-being.

These techniques are useful tools for introducing relaxation into daily life since they are simple and easy to use.

Adapting Traditional Poses for Chair Yoga

Chair yoga is an outstanding modification of conventional yoga positions, making it a practical and accessible choice for everyone, particularly males over 50.

Making yoga chair-based allows participants to get the many benefits of yoga without having to get down on the floor, making it a great practice for people with restricted mobility or joint difficulties.

Begin with the sitting mountain pose: sit comfortably with your feet flat on the floor, spine straight, and hands resting on your thighs.

Engage your core muscles and take deep, focused breaths. Inhaling while arching the back and exhaling while rounding it promotes flexibility and spinal health.

Adapting warrior stances becomes simple on a chair. Warrior stance entails extending one leg forward, keeping the knee bent, while the other leg is stretched straight behind.

Chair warrior: I use a similar position, but with the chair for support, assuring stability while still receiving the advantages of the pose.

Seated twists are essential for improving spinal mobility. Begin by sitting tall, then rotate your torso to one side, using the chair's back as leverage.

This moderate twist improves flexibility and digestion, meeting the special needs of men over 50.

Chair yoga also accommodates balancing positions like tree pose. While standing on one leg might be difficult, the chair provides a dependable object for support, enabling participants to focus on increasing balance without worry of falling.

It's critical to end the session with relaxation positions, such as sitting meditation or breathing exercises.

Mindfulness activities help to reduce stress and improve mental health, which is especially good for people dealing with the problems of aging.

Adapting standard yoga positions for chair yoga provides a complete and approachable option for men over 50.

Individuals can benefit from the physical, mental, and emotional advantages of yoga while respecting their specific needs and skills by adjusting practices to accommodate a sitting position.

Chapter 3: Mind-Body Connection in Chair Yoga

Chair yoga is a transforming practice that stresses the delicate relationship between the mind and body, making it especially good for men over the age of fifty.

This gentle yoga practice adapts conventional postures to a sitting or supported position, developing a strong mind-body connection.

Chair yoga emphasizes the mind-body connection, which promotes mental clarity and emotional well-being.

Individuals can reduce stress, improve attention, and build a sense of inner peace by breathing deeply and moving mindfully.

This is especially important for men over 50, since it helps them maintain mental resilience and emotional equilibrium in the face of life's hardships.

Physically, chair yoga promotes flexibility, strength, and balance.

Gentle stretches and postures while seated can help men maintain or enhance their range of motion without putting undue pressure on their joints.

This is especially important for people over 50, as it promotes joint health and reduces the chance of injury.

The technique also promotes core strength, which is essential for maintaining stability and avoiding frequent aging concerns.

Furthermore, chair yoga is accessible and inclusive. The use of a chair as a prop adapts the exercise to different fitness levels and physical abilities. Men over 50 may find this strategy particularly intriguing because it addresses any limits while still providing considerable health advantages.

Mindfulness in chair yoga helps to reduce stress and improve general mental health.

Men over 50 frequently confront particular obstacles, and the mind-body connection developed by chair yoga offers a comprehensive approach to wellness that goes beyond the physical.

Chair yoga for men over 50 is a holistic practice that combines the mental and physical aspects.
Individuals can improve their mental and physical well-being by practicing mindful movements, breath awareness, and physical postures, resulting in a more balanced and robust attitude to aging.

Incorporating Meditation for Mental Well-being

Incorporating meditation into regular activities can greatly improve mental health, particularly for males over 50 who participate in chair yoga. Meditation is an effective stress-management technique that promotes relaxation and awareness.

The technique entails concentrating attention on the present moment, which promotes a sense of serenity and clarity.

Meditation becomes an essential component of the overall well-being journey of men over 50 who practice chair yoga.

Aside from the physical benefits of chair yoga, such as increased flexibility and balance, meditation enhances these gains by addressing mental issues. Individuals who practice meditation for merely a few minutes each day can reduce stress, improve cognitive performance, and promote emotional resilience.

To incorporate meditation easily, begin with guided sessions that focus on deep breathing and focused awareness.

 Using a comfy chair as a meditation seat complements the chair yoga environment, making it accessible to people with mobility limitations.

Progressive muscular relaxation, a method that involves regular tensing and releasing of muscle groups, can be incorporated with sitting meditation to improve relaxation even further.

Mindful breathing is a core meditation technique that helps men over 50 focus their attention and quiet their minds. The breath becomes a focus point, serving as a basic yet effective anchor for maintaining present-moment consciousness.

As people continue to practice chair yoga, integrating breath awareness with gentle movements promotes a mind-body connection and a healthy balance of physical and mental well-being.

Consistency is crucial to reaping the full advantages of meditation. Short meditation sessions before or after chair yoga help to build a pattern, which contributes to long-term mental clarity and emotional balance.

Men over the age of 50 can benefit from enhanced mental health thanks to this comprehensive approach, which fosters a sense of general vigor and resilience in their everyday lives.

Stress Reduction and Mindful Relaxation

Stress reduction and mindful relaxation are critical components of sustaining overall well-being, especially for men over 50, who may face specific problems associated with aging. Incorporating chair yoga into their regimen may be a very beneficial method.

Chair yoga provides a mild approach to physical activity, making it suitable for people of all fitness levels.

The practice consists of modified yoga positions performed while seated or supported by a chair, with the goal of increasing flexibility, balance, and strength.

For men over 50, this is especially important since it tackles typical age-related concerns such as joint stiffness and decreased mobility.

Mindful relaxation practices, such as deep breathing and meditation, enhance chair yoga by promoting mental peace.

Deep breathing exercises induce a soothing reaction in the neurological system, minimizing the effects of stress hormones.

Combining these strategies with chair yoga results in a comprehensive strategy that not only improves physical health but also fosters mental resilience.

Consistency is essential. A consistent regimen of chair yoga and focused relaxation can help reduce stress over time.

Men over 50 may find it advantageous to include these techniques into their daily routine, even if only for a short time.

This consistent commitment can result in better sleep, less physical stress, and enhanced cognitive function.

Additionally, chair yoga fosters a sense of camaraderie and support. Joining a chair yoga class or participating in virtual sessions helps men over 50 interact with others who have similar obstacles.

This social element improves mental health by minimizing feelings of loneliness and encouraging a sense of belonging.

Chair yoga is a targeted and accessible option for guys over 50 who want to reduce stress and relax mindfully.

Individuals who embrace these practices can improve their physical and mental well-being, leading to a healthier and more balanced existence.

Enhancing Focus and Cognitive Function

Improving attention and cognitive function is critical for anyone, particularly those over 50, who wants to retain mental sharpness and general well-being.

Chair yoga promotes itself as a practical and accessible way to hone these cognitive skills.

Chair yoga for men over 50 is a customized technique that combines the advantages of conventional yoga with the comfort of sitting poses.

These mild activities stimulate improved blood flow, which improves oxygen supply to the brain. Improved oxygenation promotes cognitive function, including memory retention and mental clarity.

The emphasis on breathing methods in chair yoga promotes awareness. Mindful breathing decreases stress and improves attention.

As men age, the capacity to handle stress becomes increasingly important for cognitive health, and chair yoga offers a comprehensive approach to achieving this.

Furthermore, the physical postures in chair yoga encourage the release of endorphins, which are neurotransmitters related to mood control and cognitive performance.

These motions, designed for sitting postures, cater to the needs of older people, allowing them to participate in a low-impact yet highly effective practice.

Consistency is essential for receiving the cognitive advantages of chair yoga. Establishing a regular practice regimen promotes neuroplasticity, or the brain's ability to change and make new connections.

This adaptation is essential for preserving cognitive flexibility and resilience in the face of aging.

Incorporating chair yoga into your regular practice not only improves attention, but it also benefits general mental health.

The sense of success gained from mastering these easy positions can enhance self-esteem and confidence, hence improving cognitive function.

Chair yoga for men over 50 is a thorough way to improve attention and cognitive function. This sitting exercise provides a targeted solution for people looking to emphasize their mental health and cognitive abilities, enabling adequate oxygenation while also cultivating mindfulness and neuroplasticity.

Chapter 4: Chair Yoga Poses for Strength and Flexibility

Chair yoga is a fantastic way for those over 50, particularly males, to improve strength and flexibility in a safe and accessible setting.

Chair yoga, which is designed to suit a variety of fitness levels and physical problems, is a gentle yet effective technique to maintain overall wellness.

Seated Mountain Pose: Start with a tall spine and feet flat on the floor. Inhale, raising your arms high and activating your core muscles. This position improves posture and strengthens the spine.

Chair Cat-Cow Stretch: While sitting, arch and round your back, synchronizing movement with breathing. This dynamic stretch increases spine flexibility and decreases stiffness.

Seated Forward Bend: Hinge at the hips and reach to your toes while maintaining your back flat. This increases hamstring flexibility while stretching the lower back.

Chair Warrior positions: Take classic standing warrior positions and do them sitting. This increases leg strength and improves balance without the need to stand.

Seated Twist: Sit sideways in the chair, twist your torso to one side, and grab the backrest. This position promotes spinal mobility and massages the internal organs.

Chair Squats: Stand in front of a chair, lower yourself to a sitting posture, and then stand back up. This strengthens the legs, namely the quadriceps.

Leg lifts: Sit forward in your chair, stretch one leg at a time, and hold momentarily. This works the core and leg muscles, increasing strength and flexibility.

Chair Pigeon Pose involves crossing one ankle over the opposing knee, softly pressing on the bent knee, and sitting tall. This stretch focuses on the hips, increasing flexibility and reducing tension.

Consistent practice of these chair yoga postures for men over 50 improves physical strength and flexibility while also contributing to better balance, lower stress, and increased mental clarity.

It takes an inclusive approach to fitness, allowing anyone to enjoy the benefits of yoga without the need for a mat or considerable mobility, making it an excellent alternative for those looking for a thoughtful and accessible training program.

Building Core Strength Safely

Building core strength safely is critical, especially for men over the age of 50 who participate in chair yoga.

 A strong core increases stability, improves posture, and lowers the chance of injury. To do this safely, concentrate on controlled motions and steady growth.

Begin with simple movements like sitting twists and pelvic tilts to stimulate core muscles without effort. Incorporate breath awareness to strengthen the mind-body connection.

As you progress, incorporate increasingly difficult positions such as sitting leg raises and knee-to-chest stretches. Always emphasize good form over intensity.

Chair yoga offers good support, making it perfect for elderly people. Make sure the chair is robust and put on a non-slip surface. Maintain a comfortable seating position, feet flat on the ground. Engage the core by bringing the navel toward the spine with each movement.

Mindful growth is essential. To avoid overexertion, gradually increase exercise length and intensity. Listen to your body and adjust the positions as required. Consistency is more crucial than going too hard too quickly.

Add variation to your routine. Combine workouts that work diverse core muscles, such as the rectus abdominis, obliques, and transverse abdominis. This comprehensive method promotes balanced strength development.

Incorporate stability exercises to test the core in many planes of movement. Seated side bends and mild torso rotations can help engage and develop the core muscles.

Always warm up before starting core-focused activities. Gentle neck and shoulder rolls, as well as ankle circles, help prepare the body for movement.

 A thorough warm-up boosts blood flow to the muscles, which lowers the chance of strains.Improving core strength safely with chair yoga for men over 50 requires a cautious and attentive approach.

Prioritize perfect form, listen to your body, and improve at a speed appropriate for your fitness level. A strong core not only promotes general well-being, but it also increases the enjoyment and duration of your chair yoga practice.

Increasing Joint Flexibility and Range of Motion

Increasing joint flexibility and range of motion is critical for general health, especially as people age, particularly males over 50. Chair yoga is an excellent and accessible way to achieve these aims.

Chair yoga is a gentle yet effective way to improve joint flexibility. Incorporating sitting postures like moderate twists and side stretches promotes mobility in the spine, hips, and shoulders.

These motions are intended to progressively increase flexibility, making them excellent for anyone who has mobility issues or is new to yoga.

Furthermore, chair yoga allows you to focus on breath control and concentration. Deep, deliberate breathing during poses increases oxygen flow to the muscles and joints, which promotes suppleness.

Mindful breathing cultivates the mind-body connection, which leads to increased awareness of one's body, a sense of control over motions, and a lower chance of injury.

Adaptability is an important feature of chair yoga. Poses may be tailored to specific demands and limits, allowing men over 50 to advance at their own rate.

Consistency is essential; frequently practicing chair yoga can result in significant gains in joint flexibility and range of motion over time.

Additionally, introducing dynamic movements into chair yoga sequences might improve results. Gentle leg lifts, knee extensions, and ankle circles can all target particular joints, resulting in enhanced mobility. These exercises, when done frequently, help to enhance total joint function.

Chair yoga is an effective technique for men over 50 who want to improve joint flexibility and range of motion.

Individuals can benefit from enhanced mobility by combining sitting postures, focused breathing, adaptability, and targeted movements, all of which contribute to a healthier and more active lifestyle.

Committing to a frequent chair yoga practice allows people to age gracefully while emphasizing their physical health.

Targeted Exercises for Muscle Tone

Targeted exercises are essential for improving muscular tone, particularly for people over the age of 50 who practice chair yoga. As we get older, preserving muscle mass becomes more crucial for our general health and functionality.

Chair yoga is an accessible and effective technique for men over 50 to engage in targeted exercises that improve muscular tone and flexibility.

To improve muscular tone, chair yoga sessions should focus on specific muscle groups. Exercises that target major muscular groups, such as the legs, core, and arms, are essential.

Seated leg lifts and knee extensions can help strengthen and stabilize leg muscles. Engaging the core with sitting twists and pelvic tilts helps to tone abdominal muscles.

Chair yoga for men over 50 should involve upper-body exercises. Seated arm circles and shoulder rolls engage the shoulder muscles, increasing flexibility and tone.

Arm strengthening exercises such as bicep curls and tricep dips may be done while sitting. These targeted upper-body workouts not only help with muscular tone but also enhance general functional fitness.

Furthermore, include balance-focused poses in chair yoga practices is critical for stability and muscular activation.

Poses such as seated tree pose and seated warrior pose test balance, using numerous muscles to maintain stability, which is critical for minimizing falls and accidents in older persons.

Consistency is essential when trying for muscular tone. Men over 50 should practice chair yoga at least three times a week, progressively increasing the intensity and length as their strength improves. Furthermore, effective breathing methods should be stressed to improve relaxation and general well-being.

Targeted chair yoga exercises for men over 50 can help improve muscular tone by concentrating on specific muscle areas such as the legs, core, and upper body.

Incorporating balance-focused postures and practicing regularly will help to enhance strength, flexibility, and general health.

Chapter 5: Balancing Energy: Chair Yoga Flow

Chair yoga is a gentle yet effective technique for men over 50 to rebalance their energies and improve their general health.

This specific practice allows classic yoga positions to be performed while sitting, making it suitable for people with restricted mobility or those looking for a lower-impact workout.

To begin a chair yoga flow, choose a solid chair with no arms, sit with your feet flat on the floor, and keep your back supported.

Begin with a deep breath, inhaling through the nose and expelling through the mouth to promote relaxation. The emphasis on regulated breathing is maintained throughout the session, promoting a mind-body connection.

Begin with neck stretches, gently tilting your head from side to side and rotating it clockwise and counterclockwise.

This increases flexibility and reduces stress, which is especially good for people who spend lengthy periods of time sitting. Moving on to shoulder rolls and wrist circles helps to relieve stiffness in these regions, promoting better circulation.

The chair yoga flow focuses on sitting adaptations of fundamental yoga positions. Modified variations of warrior poses, moderate twists, and sitting forward folds work key muscle groups while improving balance and flexibility.

These positions help to improve posture, which is essential for preserving spinal health, especially in older people.

Chair yoga also focuses on the lower body with leg lifts and ankle circles. These motions increase circulation, decrease stiffness, and improve joint mobility.

As participants advance, adding resistance bands or tiny weights can provide an additional challenge, increasing strength without placing too much strain on joints.

The program ends with a guided relaxation, which allows participants to center themselves and reap the physical and mental benefits of the exercise.

Regular chair yoga practice may boost overall energy levels, reduce stress, and improve mood, all of which are important components of maintaining a healthy and active lifestyle for men over the age of 50.

Chair yoga allows you to balance your energies in a way that is more than simply a physical exercise.

Flowing Sequences for a Gentle Workout

Flowing sequences for a mild workout, particularly designed for men over 50 who participate in chair yoga, provide a comprehensive approach to physical health.

These sequences emphasize flexibility, movement, and relaxation, recognizing the special demands of this group.

Beginning with deep breathing techniques, participants are urged to center themselves, which promotes awareness and reduces stress.

Gentle neck stretches relieve stress that accumulates from sedentary lifestyles, improving mobility and decreasing stiffness.

Moving on to the upper body, fluid arm exercises improve flexibility and relieve stiffness caused by extended sitting. Incorporating circular movements activates the shoulder joints and increases range of motion. Seated twists are effortlessly incorporated, increasing spinal flexibility and improving digestion.

Moving on to the lower body, leg lifts and ankle rolls target often-overlooked muscle groups, treating concerns including joint stiffness and improving circulation.

Gentle knee-to-chest stretches relieve lower back pain while promoting relaxation and release.

The flowing patterns have a consistent speed, minimizing sudden movements that might strain muscles or joints. This stepwise approach offers a safe and successful workout while taking into account the special needs of men over 50.

The emphasis on fluidity fosters a feeling of rhythm, making the workout fun and accessible.The addition of chair support guarantees stability, allowing people of all fitness levels to engage comfortably.

Furthermore, the sitting nature of these exercises makes them perfect for those with mobility issues, making them an accessible alternative for a wide range of people.

Finishing the session with relaxation positions, such as sitting meditation or guided breathing exercises, allows participants to decompress mentally and physically.

These sequences increase not just flexibility and mobility, but also general well-being, making them an important part of a comprehensive fitness program for men over 50 who practice chair yoga.

Chair Sun Salutations for Vitality

Chair Sun Salutations are a revitalizing exercise designed specifically for men over 50, increasing energy and general well-being.

This sitting version of conventional Sun Salutations offers a gentle yet effective technique to improve flexibility, strength, and awareness without the use of a yoga mat or complicated positions.

The routine begins with focused breathing, which grounds practitioners in the present moment.

Men over the age of 50 can take deep, purposeful breaths while seated comfortably in a chair, developing a link between breathing and action. This breath awareness lays the groundwork for a comprehensive practice that promotes relaxation and mental clarity.

The flowing motions of Chair Sun Salutations are intended to improve joint mobility and flexibility.

 Gentle stretches focus on important regions such as the spine, shoulders, and hips, relieving stiffness that is typically linked with age.

These flowing motions are accessible and adaptive, providing a safe and pleasurable experience for people of all fitness levels.

As the pattern advances, it smoothly incorporates strength-building elements. Modified chair poses, such as the sitting mountain pose and chair warrior, work core muscles and increase stability.

This personalized approach addresses the special needs of men over 50, promoting muscular strength and balance to support everyday activities while lowering the risk of injury.

Chair Sun Salutations promote joint health. The regulated, rhythmic motions promote a full range of motion, increasing joint flexibility while reducing pain.

This is especially advantageous for males of this age range since it tackles typical issues such as arthritis and joint stiffness.

Mindfulness is a major concept throughout the practice. Practitioners develop a sense of inner awareness and mental clarity by focusing on the breath and making deliberate movements.

This mind-body link not only helps to reduce stress, but it also improves general health.

Chair Sun Salutations for Men Over 50 offer a complete and accessible approach to yoga. This sitting practice integrates breath awareness, flexibility, strength, and mindfulness, providing a comprehensive approach to increasing energy and promoting a healthier, more active lifestyle.

Energizing the Body through Breath and Movement

Energizing the body via breath and movement is an important part of maintaining overall well-being, especially for men over 50 who participate in chair yoga.

This type of exercise smoothly integrates the advantages of regulated breathing methods with moderate movements, providing a comprehensive approach to improving physical and mental health.

Chair yoga is a comfortable and accessible option for men over 50 to include exercise into their daily routine, accommodating a variety of fitness levels and physical restrictions.

The practice frequently begins with conscious breathing techniques that emphasize deep inhalations and exhalations. This focused breathwork not only oxygenates the body but also promotes relaxation, stress reduction, and mental clarity.

Incorporating mild motions while sitting in a chair enhances the invigorating benefits. These motions range from simple stretches to more dynamic workouts that target various muscle groups and increase flexibility.

The emphasis on perfect posture in chair yoga helps men over 50 improve their balance and core strength, both of which are important for maintaining stability and preventing injuries.

One of the primary benefits of chair yoga is the potential to improve circulation. The combination of breath control and activity increases blood flow, which promotes cardiovascular health and general vigor.

Improved circulation leads to greater tissue oxygenation, which helps reduce the muscular stiffness and joint pain that come with aging.

As men mature, joint flexibility becomes increasingly important. Chair yoga is a moderate way to address this issue, encouraging flexibility in movement and reducing stiffness.

Regular practice helps to enhance range of motion, lower the chance of injury, and improve general mobility.

Chair yoga for men over 50 provides a holistic method for revitalizing the body via deliberate breathing and gentle movements.

This holistic technique promotes physical well-being by enhancing flexibility, balance, circulation, and joint function. Including chair yoga in your practice not only encourages a more invigorated body but also leads to a greater sense of energy and well-being.

Chapter 6: Chair Yoga for Common Health Concerns

Chair yoga is a versatile and accessible type of exercise that is excellent for those with common health issues, particularly males over 50.

This low-impact practice allows classic yoga postures to be performed while sitting or supported by a chair, making it appropriate for anyone with restricted mobility or specific health conditions.

Chair yoga tackles a variety of health conditions that men over 50 frequently experience as they age. For starters, it improves joint flexibility and range of motion, which are essential for preserving mobility and avoiding stiffness.

The gentle motions assist to lubricate the joints, minimizing the pain associated with illnesses such as arthritis.

Furthermore, chair yoga improves balance and stability, lowering the risk of falls, a major issue for older persons.

It focuses on core muscles, increasing general stability and confidence in daily tasks. This is especially important for males over 50, who may notice a steady loss in balance-related skills.

The approach also emphasizes respiratory health. Controlled breathing techniques in chair yoga improve lung capacity and oxygenation, which benefits those with respiratory diseases or who are at risk of cardiovascular problems.

Improved circulation promotes heart health, which is especially important for the elderly.

Additionally, chair yoga helps to reduce tension. Men over the age of 50 frequently experience higher stress owing to a variety of life circumstances.

Chair yoga incorporates mindfulness and relaxation practices, which assist to manage stress and promote mental well-being.

Furthermore, the adjustability of chair yoga makes it appropriate for people recuperating from injuries or managing chronic diseases.

It offers a moderate yet efficient way to keep physically active without increasing pre-existing health conditions.

Chair yoga emerges as a holistic solution for men over 50, addressing joint flexibility, balance, lung health, stress reduction, and adaptation to a variety of medical issues.

This accessible approach enables people to focus their well-being and live an active lifestyle, resulting in a happier and more happy existence throughout their elderly years.

Alleviating Back Pain and Discomfort

Relief of back pain and stiffness is critical for men over 50 who want to live a healthy and active lifestyle. Chair yoga is an increasingly popular and successful practice.

This low-impact form of exercise provides a complete approach to treating back pain while being accessible to people of all fitness levels.

Chair yoga consists of mild stretches and motions that may be done while seated. These exercises are designed to improve flexibility, strengthen core muscles, and promote good posture, all of which are important in the treatment of back pain.

Chair yoga is a practical and reasonable alternative for men over the age of 50 who may be tight and have limited flexibility.

Mindful breathing is an important part of chair yoga for back pain alleviation. Deep, regulated breathing relaxes stiff muscles and improves the overall efficiency of the activities.

This thoughtful approach not only alleviates physical suffering but also enhances mental health by lowering stress, which can lead to back pain.

Regular chair yoga practices promote blood circulation, which is necessary for spinal repair and nourishment.

The mild motions done while seated cause the production of endorphins, which promote a sensation of well-being and naturally alleviate suffering.

Furthermore, chair yoga accommodates those with restricted mobility, making it an inclusive choice for people who may find conventional yoga difficult.

When implementing chair yoga into a back pain relief practice, it is critical to maintain consistency. Setting aside time each day or week for these exercises might help you progressively gain strength and flexibility.

Additionally, men over the age of 50 should contact a healthcare practitioner before beginning any new fitness plan to verify it is appropriate for their specific health needs.

Chair yoga stands out as an efficient and accessible method for relieving back pain and suffering, particularly for men over 50.

Its mix of mild stretches, focused breathing, and flexibility makes it an effective tool for improving spine health and general well-being.

Managing Arthritis with Gentle Exercises

Gentle activities, particularly chair yoga, can help men over 50 manage their arthritis and relieve joint pain and stiffness.

Arthritis, a prevalent illness among older people, can have a substantial impact on mobility and general well-being.

Gentle workouts are essential for preserving joint flexibility, decreasing inflammation, and increasing muscular strength.

Chair yoga is a practical solution for people with arthritis, providing a low-impact option that is accessible to people of all fitness levels. Chair yoga's sitting postures and regulated movements are mild on the joints, making it an excellent alternative for men over 50 who suffer from arthritic symptoms. This type of exercise improves joint range of motion and flexibility while minimizing stress on sensitive regions.

Chair yoga for arthritis management consists of sitting positions and regulated breathing techniques.

These motions improve blood circulation, which promotes nutrition supply to the joints and aids in the clearance of pollutants.

Furthermore, chair yoga's emphasis on mindfulness and relaxation can help to reduce stress, which has been shown to increase arthritic symptoms.

It is critical for males over 50 to practice chair yoga consistently and moderately. Regular practice, even for short periods of time, can progressively improve strength and flexibility. Warm-up activities before chair yoga sessions are vital for preparing the body for movement and lowering the chance of injury.

Consulting with a healthcare expert or a certified yoga instructor may give specific direction and ensure that exercises are matched to each individual's requirements and limits.

Incorporating chair yoga into one's everyday practice enables people to take an active part in controlling arthritis. It supports other parts of arthritis treatment, such as medication and lifestyle changes.

Gentle activities such as chair yoga can help men over 50 improve joint function, reduce discomfort, and improve their general quality of life.

Enhancing Circulation and Heart Health

Improving circulation and heart health is critical for general wellness, especially as people age.

For men over the age of 50, including chair yoga into their regimen can be a highly effective and accessible strategy to reach these goals.

Chair yoga is a low-impact workout alternative suitable for people of all fitness levels and physical constraints. Chair yoga's gentle motions and stretches boost blood flow throughout the body, which helps to improve circulation.

Improved circulation, in turn, promotes improved oxygenation of tissues and organs, lowering the risk of cardiovascular disease.

Regular chair yoga practice might also improve heart health. Yoga's regulated breathing methods help regulate blood pressure, lowering strain on the heart.

Furthermore, the mild nature of chair yoga reduces the danger of overexertion, making it a suitable option for people with pre-existing cardiac issues.

Furthermore, chair yoga improves flexibility and strength, both of which are necessary for cardiovascular health.

Muscle strengthening, particularly in the lower body, benefits the heart by increasing its ability to pump blood more efficiently.

Improved flexibility leads to healthier circulation by allowing blood vessels to operate properly, lowering the risk of arterial stiffness caused by age.

Consistency is essential for maximizing the advantages of chair yoga for heart health. Short, everyday workouts can help to progressively improve endurance, stamina, and general cardiovascular health.

It is crucial to remember that chair yoga is more than just physical exercise; it also promotes stress reduction and mental well-being, both of which have an indirect impact on heart health.

Chair yoga for men over 50 provides a comprehensive approach to improving circulation and heart health.

Its mix of moderate movements, regulated breathing, and emphasis on overall fitness makes it an accessible and successful option for anyone looking to promote cardiovascular well-being in their older years.

Chapter 7: Personalizing Your Chair Yoga Practice

Personalizing your chair yoga practice is essential, particularly for men over 50 who want specialized routines that address their specific demands and physical circumstances. To reap the full advantages of chair yoga, customisation is essential.

Begin by recognizing your body's limitations and strengths. Men over the age of 50 frequently experience joint problems and limited flexibility.

Modify standard chair yoga postures to address these difficulties. To preserve joints, instead of deep knee bends, use milder exercises. Tailoring your practice to target particular areas of discomfort leads to a safer and more pleasurable experience.

Consider doing targeted stretches to increase flexibility. Concentrate on regions prone to stiffness, such as the hips, lower back, and shoulders. Gentle twists and hip-opening exercises help reduce tension and increase range of motion.

Emphasizing flexibility in your chair yoga program helps to retain general mobility, which is a typical worry for men as they age.

In addition, engage in strength-building workouts to prevent muscle loss caused by aging.

 Use the chair to provide support during leg lifts, sitting squats, and arm workouts. This not only builds muscles but also improves balance, which is an important part of maintaining stability and avoiding falls.

Breathwork is another important aspect of chair yoga. Add mindful breathing methods to your practice to make it more personalized. Deep belly breathing can help you relax and reduce tension. Tailoring your breathwork to your own requirements can help you achieve better mental health, which is especially important for men dealing with the challenges of aging.

Finally, customize your chair yoga program by setting achievable objectives. Set attainable goals and measure your progress.

Having specific goals, whether they be for more flexibility, enhanced balance, or lower stress, boosts motivation and provides a sense of achievement.

Personalizing chair yoga for men over 50 entails modifying postures, stressing flexibility and strength, including mindful breathwork, and creating achievable goals. Tailoring your practice to your specific requirements allows you to gain the full advantages of chair yoga, which promotes physical and mental well-being as you age.

Creating Customized Routines for Individual Needs

Developing personalized routines for people, particularly those tailored to their specific demands, is critical for maximizing the advantages of any fitness plan.

This idea is especially important when contemplating chair yoga for men over 50.

Creating a routine that is tailored to their physical condition, preferences, and general well-being is critical for a comprehensive and successful practice.

To begin, evaluate the individual's health and any unique concerns or limits. This may include speaking with a healthcare practitioner to confirm that the selected regimen is safe and appropriate. Understanding joint flexibility, muscular strength, and current medical issues will help guide the customisation process.

In chair yoga, adaptability is essential. Begin with easy warm-up movements that increase blood flow and flexibility. Incorporate joint mobility exercises, focusing on regions of stiffness that are frequent in older persons.

Controlled breathing throughout the routine not only promotes relaxation but also helps to improve lung capacity and circulation.

The program should advance gradually, using a variety of sitting positions that enhance balance, strength, and flexibility. Poses such as sitting mountain position, moderate twists, and forward bends might be useful.

Adjust the difficulty to the practitioner's comfort level, and progressively add more hard postures as confidence and strength grow.

Chair yoga's mental and emotional advantages can be enhanced by including mindfulness and meditation techniques.

Encourage them to focus on the present moment, which will help them relax and reduce tension. Mindful breathing techniques can improve your general well-being.

Reassess the routine on a regular basis and alter it as appropriate, taking into account any health gains or changes.

Flexibility is essential in altering the routine to changing demands, resulting in a sustainable and pleasurable practice.

Developing a personalized chair yoga regimen for men over 50 requires careful consideration of their health, interests, and goals. A customized and successful workout routine can enhance physical, mental, and emotional well-being by being tailored to individual needs and constantly adapted over time.

Integrating Chair Yoga into Daily Life

Chair yoga is a simple and accessible approach for men over 50 to include light exercise and mindfulness into their everyday routines.

Maintaining flexibility, balance, and mental well-being becomes increasingly important as we age, and chair yoga efficiently meets these demands.

Start your chair yoga practice with sitting warm-up activities, including mild neck and shoulder stretches.

Use regulated breathing to improve relaxation and concentration. These exercises may be easily included in your morning or evening routine, providing a great start or end to your day.

At work, practice chair yoga by taking brief pauses to stretch and relieve stress. Simple sitting postures and twists can reduce stiffness and enhance circulation, resulting in greater productivity and less stress.

Incorporating chair yoga into your workplace also encourages improved posture, which may help ease back discomfort caused by extended sitting.

Consider enrolling in a chair yoga session tailored particularly for guys over the age of 50.
Experienced teachers may lead you through a range of postures tailored to your age group's specific needs, building a friendly community of like-minded people.

This social aspect provides a sense of camaraderie, making the exercise more fun and inspiring.

Chair yoga is adjustable to different fitness levels and physical conditions, making it a good choice for anyone who has restricted mobility or is recuperating from an injury. Accept changes and go at your own speed to provide a safe and sustainable practice.

Aside from the physical benefits, chair yoga offers an excellent chance for mental relaxation and stress reduction.

Incorporate mindfulness practices, such as meditation and deep breathing, into your daily routine to improve attention and emotional well-being.

Men over the age of 50 can benefit from including chair yoga in their everyday lives. Its versatility, ease, and multiple advantages make it an effective option for improving flexibility, balance, and general well-being.

Begin with tiny, steady steps and discover the benefits of chair yoga for your physical and emotional wellness.

Staying Consistent and Adapting Over Time

Consistency and adaptation are crucial factors in developing and maintaining a healthy lifestyle, particularly for men over the age of 50 who practice chair yoga.

Consistency with a chair yoga exercise is essential for enjoying the long-term advantages of increased flexibility, better posture, and general well-being.

Establishing a regular practice, even if it is only for a few minutes every day, helps to gradually but steadily enhance physical and mental health.

Adapting over time is equally crucial. Men's bodies vary as they age, and so do their exercise demands. The chair yoga regimen must be modified to meet these changes, ensuring that the movements remain effective and safe. This adaptability may include altering the intensity of postures, introducing variants to treat particular issues such as joint stiffness or muscle tightness, and being aware of personal limitations.

Consistency and adaptation go hand in hand. Consistent practice establishes a foundation of strength and flexibility, whereas adaptability allows for tailored modifications to match the specific needs of an individual's body.

This combination not only improves physical health but also increases mental resilience. Chair yoga becomes a tool not just for physical fitness, but also for dealing with the obstacles that age might bring.

Furthermore, consistency extends beyond the yoga mat. A holistic approach to health includes eating a well-balanced diet, staying hydrated, and getting enough rest. Adapting food choices to suit increasing nutritional demands and altering sleep habits to aid recuperation are critical concerns for men over 50.

Chair yoga for men over 50 is based on the concepts of consistency and gradual adaptation.

A dedication to regular practice, along with a readiness to adapt the routine as needed, is the foundation of a healthy and sustainable approach to fitness. This approach not only promotes physical well-being but also enables people to face the aging process with fortitude and grace.

CONCLUSION

Yoga emerges as a comprehensive and helpful practice for men over 50, providing several physical, mental, and emotional benefits. As people get older, they realize how important it is to retain flexibility, balance, and general health.

Yoga proved to be a versatile option, meeting the specific demands of this group. Yoga positions are mild yet helpful in improving joint mobility and muscular flexibility, treating typical age-related ailments including arthritis and stiffness.

Beyond the physical sphere, yoga promotes mental resilience and emotional balance. The contemplative features of yoga create a peaceful environment for men over 50 to manage stress, improve attention, and build awareness.

This is especially important in an age group that frequently deals with life transitions, retirement, and potential health difficulties.

Yoga's versatility allows people to modify their practice to suit their own fitness levels and health concerns, providing inclusion for everyone.

Yoga courses frequently include a sense of community, which adds a vital social component to the practice.

 Men over 50 gain not just from physical and mental health benefits but also from the companionship produced by yoga clubs.

Yoga, being a low-impact, accessible exercise, becomes a sustainable lifestyle choice for this generation, encouraging longevity, vigor, and a harmonious body-mind balance.

Embracing yoga in your senior years may be a transforming experience, improving the overall quality of life for men facing the specific obstacles of aging.

THANK YOU PAGE

Thank you for selecting this book. Your support is really appreciated. Similarly, I am grateful for the purchase of this book.

Your input is valuable; please share your ideas in a review. It serves as a reference for future improvements. Enjoy reading and utilizing it!